Vitamin D:

# Vitamin D Deficiency and Prevention of Chronic Diseases

By Ryan Seager

***

# Vitamin D:

# Vitamin D Deficiency and Prevention of Chronic Diseases

By Ryan Seager © 2014 All Rights Reserved Worldwide

\*\*\*

# Table of Contents

# Introduction

Vitamin D is known as the 'sunshine vitamin'. Part of our skin as humans is specifically designed to produce Vitamin D from being exposed to the UV rays of the sun. The chemical interaction that occurs between chemicals in the skin and UV rays produces Vitamin D3 also known as cholecalciferol. Your skin is very efficient at producing Vitamin D; in fact after about 20 minutes of sun exposure (or about 1 hour for dark skinned individuals) your body will reach an equilibrium level of Vitamin D and stop producing any excess.

Throughout history humans have lived with exposure to the Sun as a normal part of day-to-day life. It is only in recent times that people have begun to avoid sun exposure, sometimes avoiding any and all contact with the solar rays that are known to induce the production of Vitamin D. Because of these and other lifestyle changes; that is, spending all day indoors or working in an office for example, almost anyone can be at risk of having a vitamin D deficiency.

## Why should I care about Vitamin D deficiency?

Vitamin D deficiency has been associated with rickets (osteomalacia) for some time. That is the softening of the bones, especially in children; causing them to become bowlegged. But that is only one of the effects; a vitamin D deficiency is also associated with: diabetes, multiple sclerosis, rheumatoid arthritis, infectious diseases, heart disease and cancer.

The question arises, if a person takes Vitamin D supplements, is it the same as the vitamin D that is produced by the sun? Doctors and scientists are not sure whether the effect on the body is precisely the same – when your body produces vitamin D from sun exposure, the skin is simultaneously producing additional photo-products and chemicals that may complement the production of vitamin D in ways that are not fully understood yet. In spite of this dilemma, doctors do know that Vitamin D supplementation if effective in preventive the most obvious signs of vitamin D deficiency such as rickets (Osteomalacia).

The earliest successful treatment for rickets was carried out in 1919 by a fellow by the name of Kurt Huldschinsky; he was able to cure children of rickets by exposing them to light from a mercury vapor lamp. His treatment was very controversial at the time but was also vital since rickets was an epidemic amongst children at that time in history. (Just imagine that in 1889 in the city of Boston, 80% of infants suffered from rickets) Soon after, in 1921, it was demonstrated that similar results could be obtained by exposure to sunlight.

In 1931 the U.S. even issued guidelines recommending parents to exposure their children to sunlight. I remember myself as a child, my mother used to tell me and brothers to go outside and play 'bare-chested' in the summer months.

Eventually the associated research of that time led to the discovery of the relationship between rickets and Vitamin D.

Since the early 1900's and through an understanding of the benefits of vitamin D, rickets is now almost unheard of in modern society. Scientists discovered that if they irradiated food; that is, expose food to UV rays, it would cause the production of Vitamin D in the food. They started doing this to milk and since then rickets was eradicated as a health problem. On a side note, Quaker Oats became the first company to add Vitamin D to its breakfast cereal in 1927.

More recent developments, however, have reversed the endorsement of sun exposure and that has mostly been due to the influence of dermatology associations who link sun exposure to skin cancer. Today, it is never recommended to get direct sun exposure; instead people are strongly encouraged to use sunscreen to prevent any exposure to UV rays.

Because rickets is no longer a huge health concern, and because vitamin D has been added to milk, the concern about sufficient levels of vitamin D in one's diet has more or less fallen off the radar. Yet Vitamin D is still and has always been a vital component for bone health. Especially in infants and children, a vitamin D deficiency during the developmental years can results in serious health problems for the rest of their lives. And serious cases of rickets still crop up now and again in North America, about a dozen cases per year in major cities.

The UK Telegraph also reported: "Between 1998 and 2011, the number of cases of rickets admitted to hospital each year increased more than five-fold, from 147 to 762." So for a disease that was essentially eradicated, you can see that unless people are vigilant, a vitamin D deficiency can occur resulting in serious consequences.

Sometimes these modern day cases of rickets are due to breastfeeding mothers being advised by their doctors that breast milk provides all the nutrients a baby needs. The fact of the matter is that breast milk is low in vitamin D, only about 25 IU/L (25 international units per litre). The recommended daily allowance of vitamin D is 600 IU. (600 international units) and for pregnant women, the recommended amount should be 1000 IU per day. According to Dr. Holick at the Boston University School of Medicine, pregnant women would need to take 4000 to 6000 IU of vitamin D per day to ensure that their breast milk contains enough vitamin D for the baby.

The American Academy of Pediatrics now recommends that babies need 400 IU of vitamin D per day for the first year of life.

## Getting Vitamin D from Food

Many people remember their parents giving them cod liver oil when they were children. This practice has for the most part fallen out of fashion even though it was a good way to get more vitamin D into the diet. Unfortunately most people do not like the taste of cod liver oil. Even the capsules can leave a bad taste after they dissolve in the stomach.

You can also get good quantities of vitamin D from oily fish such as salmon, tuna, mackerel and sardines. A 3.5 oz serving of these types of fish provide about 500 IU of Vitamin D.

You can also get vitamin D from eggs (about 40 IU per egg) and fortified milk.(one eight ounce glass of milk has about 120 IU of vitamin D) Fortified milk has vitamin D2 added; which is not as readily used by the body as Vitamin D3. There is a food chart included in the section on Vitamin D and Cancer and more details about the differences between vitamin D2 and vitamin D3 will also be covered.

## Different types of Vitamin D

You will often find Vitamin D supplements come in different forms. Vitamin D3 is also known as choleciferol, this form of vitamin D is readily used by the body. This type of vitamin D is the kind that is produced in the skin from sun exposure and it is also manufactured from animal sources.

There is also Vitamin D2, known as ergocalciferol which is more common but is slightly harder for the body to process. This is the type of Vitamin D that is added to fortified milk. Vitamin D2 is produced from plants and fungi. The exact chemical differences will be covered in a later section of this book.

Studies have shown that Vitamin D3 is only 30% effective at being absorbed and processed by the body than Vitamin D2.

An independent study by Dr, Holick was conducted where he gave healthy adults 1000 IU of Vitamin D2 per day or 1000 IU of Vitamin D3 per day for three months. The study was conducted at the end of the summer so that sunlight exposure would not influence the results. The results showed only a small marginal better performance of D3 raising blood levels of vitamin D over D2. After many tests mixing the amounts and comparing, it was determined that the difference between Vitamin D2 and Vitamin D3 is not significant.

A regimen of 1000 IU per day in additional to getting a monthly boost of a high dosage of Vitamin D would be effective to maintain a healthy level of Vitamin D in your body. For example, **taking a once-a-day supplement of 1000 IU of vitamin D and then getting 15 to 30 minutes of sun exposure once a week or once every two weeks would be an excellent way to maintain healthy levels of Vitamin D in your body.**

## Vitamin D from the Sun

You might think that you can make sufficient vitamin D from the sun but according to some independent studies, you cannot make any Vitamin D at all during the months of November through February if you are anywhere above about 35 degrees latitude north. That is at the level of latitude equal to Atlanta, Georgia. If you live in a place like New York for example, you would not be able to make any vitamin D from the sun from about mid October to about early April.

Of course if you live in Florida, your skin could produce Vitamin D all year long. But now you have to ask the question of the effect of sunscreen. Almost everyone today uses sunscreen. If you use a sunscreen with an SPF of 15; this will reduce the ability of your skin to make vitamin D by about 95 to 99%. This makes sense because SPF sunscreen reduces the ability of UVB rays to affect your skin and it is these rays that induce the production of vitamin D in your body.

A good dose of sun exposure (without using sunscreen of course) and not to the point of burning; say a fifteen to thirty minute tanning session can produce 10,000 to 20,000 IU of Vitamin D for the individual and this level of production is seen over the span of about 24 hours after sun exposure.

## Vitamin D production and aging

As we age, our ability to produce Vitamin D also grows less. A seventy year old has about 75% less ability to produce vitamin D than a twenty year old. However, studies have shown that for the elderly, even just 15 to 30 minutes exposure of their arms and legs just twice or three times per week makes a considerable difference in raising the blood levels of vitamin D for these seniors.[1]

---

[1] According to research conducted by Bone Research Laboratory, Boston University School of Medicine

## Vitamin D Deficiency Symptoms

Vitamin D deficiency often goes undetected because the symptoms can be associated with other conditions. People have reported having difficulty sleeping, they have a general feeling of tiredness or even depression. A common symptom is muscle cramps or muscle aches and pains. Some have reported sore fingers especially at the last knuckle at the extremities of the fingers; they may find it painful to shake hands. Some of the symptoms are often associated with osteoporosis or arthritis and because Vitamin D helps with calcium absorption, there may be some overlap with these conditions and symptoms.

Other reported symptoms include flu-like aches and pains, psoriasis and periodontal disease. There is a separate section about psoriasis later in this book and the appendixes also have detailed examination of specific symptom; especially the severe cases of extreme vitamin D deficiency that lead to bone deformation.

## Obesity and Vitamin D deficiency

Experiments were conducted wherein individuals were given 50,000 IU of Vitamin D2; they compared the resulting blood levels of those with average weight with those who were obese and the obese individuals had 55% less vitamin D in their blood. This makes sense because vitamin D is fat soluble and will be absorbed by the excess fat in obese individuals. Therefore obese people likely need 2 to 3 times more vitamin D in their diet to maintain healthy levels of vitamin D. This could be as much as 50,000 IU of vitamin D per week.

In 2012 the American Journal of Epidemiology reported an analysis of data from 2500 Norwegian adults that showed that obesity and vitamin D levels are directly related; in other words obese individuals are much more likely to be vitamin D deficient that those with a healthy body mass index.

Even more importantly from this same study, it was discovered that normal weight individuals with low vitamin D levels are more likely to develop obesity over time than individuals with healthy levels of vitamin D. In other words, healthy levels of vitamin D can help to **prevent** becoming overweight and obesity. There was <u>no</u> <u>evidence</u> from this study that Vitamin D supplementation can cause weight loss however there are anecdotal cases of individuals who have reported weight loss by taking large doses of vitamin D.

You can expect more research to continue in this area in the near future since the demand for weight loss solutions are obviously so important in today's health conscious and body conscious society.

# Recommendations from Dietary Researchers

Michael Holick, the Director of the Vitamin D Skin and Bone Research Laboratory in Boston recommends 5 to 15 minutes of direct sunlight two or three times per week, exposing the arms and legs prior to applying sunscreen. Once this amount of sun exposure is reached, you can apply sunscreen or cover up the skin with clothing.

Melanin is efficient as a natural sunscreen in blocking UV rays so black individuals would need 5 to 10 times the amount of sun exposure to get the same vitamin D benefit as Caucasians.

As far as the current recommended Adequate Intake (AI) levels of Vitamin D are concerned, they are as follows:

Age 0 to 50 years old: 200 IU per day

Age 50 to 70 years old: 400 IU per day

Age 70 and above: 600 IU per day

The National Osteoporosis Foundation recommends a daily intake of 800 to 1000 IU of Vitamin D per day for all adults.

## More Details on Vitamin D Deficiency

It is estimated that as much as 50% of the population may be vitamin D deficient. Now this vitamin D deficiency can lead to osteoporosis but most people are not diagnosed with this until they have an actual bone fracture. Vitamin D deficiency also leads to osteomalacia (inadequate mineralization in the bones) and is often diagnosed as fibromyalgia. This results in muscle aches and pains and sore joints and even depression. By improving the intake of vitamin D, these patients will experience an improvement in well being and a decrease in symptoms after about six months so it does take time to reverse a condition of vitamin D deficiency.

There have been cases of people that are so sore in their bones that they cannot sit down comfortably – again the cause was linked to vitamin D deficiency and the pain and discomfort was able to be reversed over time by increasing vitamin D intake which in turn had the effect of increasing the bone density of the individual.

Many people visit doctor complaining of bone pain, lower back pain (lumbar pain) accompanied with depression and are given pain killers and sent home. All the while they do not have any idea that they are vitamin D deficient. Some people have even been misdiagnosed with ALS (Arterial Lateral Sclerosis) when in fact they were simply vitamin D deficient.

Some studies have linked vitamin D deficiency with Parkinson's disease and dementia but those results are still inconclusive or are in process of being corroborated at this point.

Vitamin D receptors are actually in the skeletal muscle; so not surprisingly an increase in vitamin D levels correlates to stronger and more coordinated muscle function.

Vitamin D and calcium naturally go together because Vitamin D is needed to allow your body to absorb the calcium. Taking calcium and vitamin D together will help strengthen bones and help to prevent hip fractures in the elderly.

## Treating Vitamin D Deficiency

The first thing that comes to mind for treating Vitamin D deficiency is to take a multi-vitamin. That is a good start but unfortunately most multi-vitamins only contain 400 IU of vitamin D. It is not a good idea to take more than one multi-vitamin because there may be negative effects from taking too much of the other ingredients; for example taking more than one multi-vitamin would result in excessive consumption of vitamin A. The same is true if taking cod-liver oil. A tablet of cod-liver oil gives you 200 IU of Vitamin D but it also gives you 2500 IU of vitamin A.

It is better to take a supplement of Vitamin D that has no other ingredients. Examples of some good vitamin D supplements are given in the section on retail products.

Cases of Vitamin D deficiency have been treated with massive doses of Vitamin D with no ill effects; for example patients were given 50,000 IU once a week for eight weeks to bring up their blood levels. Furthermore, a group of patients were given 50,000 IU of D2 every other week for 6 years, and there was no excessive build up, nor toxicity.

## Vitamin D Toxicity

There is little to no danger of Vitamin D toxicity even at a dosage of 10,000 IU per day. If a person took, say, 50,000 IU per day then yes, they would likely quickly get Vitamin D toxicity which would result in excess calcium build up and possible kidney damage. As far as the recommend dosage of 1000 IU per day, there is no danger of building up excess Vitamin D in the blood. Also the human skin is very efficient at processing UV rays so there is also no danger of excessive Vitamin D build up from sun exposure. If the body gets enough Vitamin D from UV rays, any excess is not processed or 'shut off' by the chemical workings within the skin.

Every cell in the human body has what is called a VDR or a 'Vitamin D Receptor'. Almost all doctors now realize how important it is to overall health whereas in the past there was a lot more worry about possible toxicity.

## Vitamin D and Cancer Prevention

As mentioned already, every cell in your body has a vitamin D receptor in it. Doctors are still not sure of all the reasons why they might be there. In 1979 Tateo Suda did a study where he took Leukemic cells and then activated the receptors of the cells with Vitamin D 3 and then discovered that they subsequently became normal.

After the study mentioned above, more research was done in the area of Vitamin D and cancer; initial efforts by researchers were often met with ridicule since they were essentially stating that sun exposure could actually reduce the risk of cancer when the prevailing sentiment was strongly opposed to this – everyone with any medical training would condemn any notion above benefits from sunlight because they were busy telling people to use sunscreen to protect themselves from skin cancer.

Early in 2014, Doctor Tannaz Armaghany gave a presentation for Westchase Clinical Associates on the topic of Vitamin D and cancer.

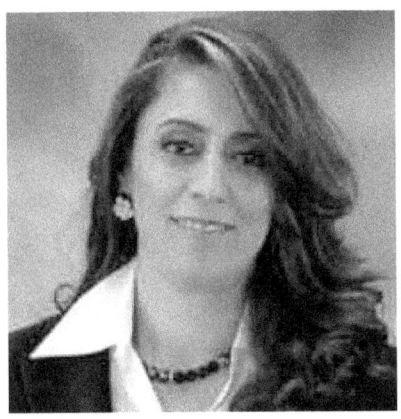

*Dr. Tannaz Armaghany*

Dr. Armaghany is a board certified hematologist and medical oncologist with special interest in Gastrointestinal oncology, Neuroendocrine tumors and integrative oncology. Here are the major details that she presented from her research and knowledge.

The most important role of vitamin D is regulating calcium and phosphorus in the blood. So vitamin D works to bring the level of calcium in the blood to normal. The other thing that it does, it has a good effect on your immune system. And, this is published in numerous papers but one important one is from Holick, in 2005, which demonstrated that, it boosts your immunity and also inhibits specific auto-immune diseases.

What type of diseases? Diabetes, MS, Arthritis, these are diseases that are categorized as auto-immune diseases. So it has a lot to do with those kinds of diseases. Vitamin D can affect insulin secretion, and it also affects some of the pancreatic cells, and that is done by the vitamin D receptor.

We can also talk about blood pressure. There was a paper by Ullah in 2010, that demonstrated how people that were under tanning beds, their vitamin D level was going up and up and up. And guess what, their blood pressure was going down. So that was an interesting result that was demonstrated. But then, more and more papers came out that showed that vitamin D deficiency is associated with high blood pressure.

Even heart failure, it's well known that people that have vitamin D problems, they can have heart failure. So people that have cardiovascular diseases like myocardial infarction or peripheral vascular diseases, most of them do have vitamin D deficiency. So we know vitamin D works in many places in the body.

As far as prevention goes, can we examine what vitamin D is able to prevent? It prevents osteoporosis, which is something that is quite common. We do dexa scans for women after 50 years old because, we know that osteoporosis is very common. So vitamin D can actually prevent that. Now we know Alzheimer's is actually also associated with vitamin D deficiency. So we also want to prevent that by making sure your vitamin D level is normal.

And again, the auto immune conditions like those mentioned already. But our topic here is about cancer, so we will focus more on that.

Basically we know that vitamin D is generated in the skin like you probably know. That is the most common way of acquiring vitamin D. So in the skin, we have seven de-hydro-cholesterols. And when the sun actually affects our skin, vitamin D3 is what is generated, in the skin. So our body can use it to actually affect our organs, what first has to happen is it changes in the liver.

So the liver actually adds an OH branch to the vitamin D molecule. And that's what we call 25-OH vitamin D3. That is the one that your doctor will check in your blood. So if you're going be checking your vitamin D level, that is what's going to be checked. That is not the most potent type of vitamin D. But it is the best test that is associated with what you eat. So we know, that is what we need to check.

But then, the OH vitamin D has to change to another molecule which is the most potent molecule, which is 25 OH vitamin D. That is the most potent and that is the one that affects all of the organs of the body.

That affects your bones and the intestines and allows your body to make your calcium and cholesterol to be absorbed.

In the pancreas it increases your insulin secretion, and that's where the diabetes problems come up. With type 1 diabetes and type 2 diabetes, you have a case of insulin levels being low. So vitamin D actually promotes insulin secretion.

In the bone marrow, it actually makes your bone marrow, it starts generating good cells in the bone marrow; so that's very important there too. So how is Vitamin D made? Well, sunlight, affects the molecule de-hydro cholesterol, and makes D3 in the skin and also basically in the liver, not only from the sun, we know that we acquire vitamin D through supplements and food sources as well.

So is you decide to go to the supplement store, there are two are very different types of vitamin D so you want to pay attention to what you are getting. These two different types do not affect the bone and the organs in the same way nor in the same potency. So let's examine that. Cholecalciferol is Vitamin D3, this is what our body is able to produce by the sun.

Ergocalciferol is Vitamin D2 and this is produced by plants. The plants actually also produce vitamin D2 from the sun. The difference between vitamin D2 and D3 is that vitamin D2 only has 40% potency. So even if you're seeing the same dose amount on the bottle, it's not going have the same affect in your body. Basically it's a kind of weaker type of vitamin D.

Now here is a map which shows the United States and which was published by W. H. O. (World Health Organization) and on it you can see a line there that shows the latitude.

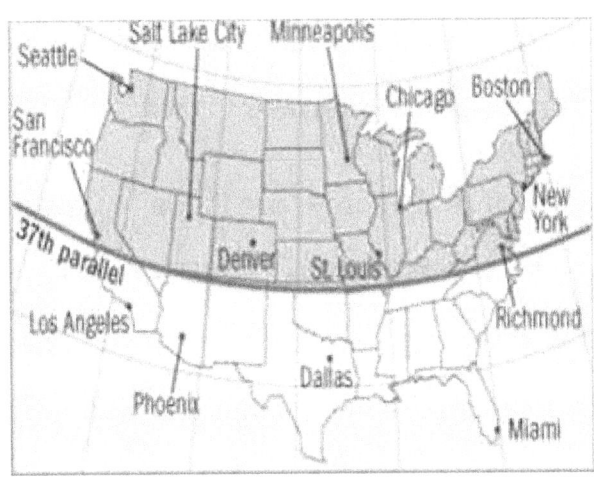

The research shows that anyone living above this latitude, above about 35 to 37 degrees latitude, they will more likely have a vitamin D deficiency.

So between the end of fall and all the way through spring, people's vitamin D levels are lower than those in the southern states. And why is that? It's because of the sun. So in the winter, in the fall, the sun rays are more oblique, they travel a longer distance through the atmosphere, so its rays get absorbed in the atmosphere. And consequently these rays don't reach the Earth's surface with the same strength as in the summer. So our skin, living in the higher latitudes, our skin is not going to be exposed to sunlight. That is why there are more people with vitamin D related problems there.

So people that are living in higher latitude states, you need to be a little more conscience about your vitamin D levels, than southerners. Do you need to check it? Of course you do. If you check your vitamin D level and it's less than 10 nanomols per litre, then you should know less than 10 is extremely deficient.

Let's mention rickets, this occurs when there is an extreme deficiency of vitamin D. We don't normally see this in the United States any more, this is usually seen in developing countries or under developed countries. This occurs when the mother had vitamin D deficiency, calcium deficiency, and that the kids are not being supplemented. So here is an extreme clinical manifestation of vitamin D deficiency.

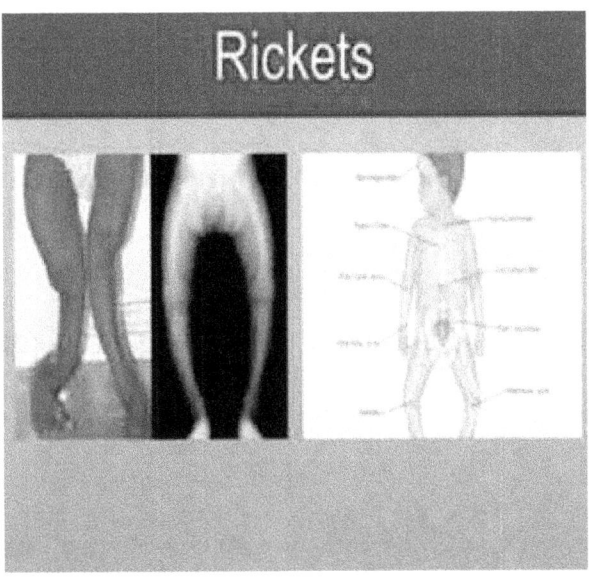

Rickets

Alright, but let's get back to our topic and what's the connection between cancer and vitamin D? Doctor Frank Garland, he's a pioneer, is the person that actually for the first time, found the connection between vitamin D deficiency and cancer; it was after years and years of research. Unfortunately, he died after being sick for a year for so at the age of 60. But he has contributed to this field a lot. And his data shows that there are at least 20 types of cancer that are associated with low vitamin D. **Now I also have to mention that, cancer is a disease that so**

**many factors are involved with so we can't say just having low vitamin D is why someone is getting cancer, but it certainly can be contributing to it and making it easier to develop that cancer.**

So he's held several seminars and talked about the role of Vitamin D in prevention of different cancers. And not only that, he showed that vitamin D deficiency or supplementing vitamin D can prevent so many devastating diseases such as diabetes, psoriasis, MS; these are things that we don't have reliable treatments for, so it's better to prevent it and not try to struggle with treating them. Even fibromyalgia, there's no treatment for this, and a lot of people suffer from it.

So, it had been 60 years without any link being made between sun exposure and cancer. It was not until the 1980s that the first hypothesis was made that there is an association and this association was seen in laboratories and in animals. In 1985, Dr. Garland, for the first time, published a paper, and talked about the

Vitamin D and cancer relationship, the deaths because of colon cancer is higher in people that are living in northern states than in southern states. So a definite connection was found.

Data was very strong for the relationship between Vitamin D deficiency and colorectal cancer and breast cancer; almost all the trials that have been done showed a very clear positive relationship. There is a suggestion of bladder cancer, gastric cancer, ovarian cancer, uterus cancer, kidney cancer, lymphomas as well. The data for prostate and pancreatic cancer was not a hundred percent matching with all the data from all the studies but still there are a lot of people who contribute vitamin D to that.

Now I mention this here because this is a study done by the government. This is the US task force, the US preventive service task force. These are people that get together and put together the guidelines for the country. And as you can imagine, they are very thorough. They have studied the association between vitamin D deficiency and bone fracture incidence and also cancer. They had 19 trials and 28 observation studies. This equates to thousands of patients that they have looked at and are trying to see if there is a connection there.

So just to give you an idea of their results, they conducted studies where they do a pool analysis which we call a meta-analysis. A pool analysis which they put all the data together and there has to be a very smart statistician to put this data together and give us the results.

If almost all of these studies as your vitamin D level in the blood is going up, your risk of colon cancer is coming down. Just look at that. And this one, and this one, and this one, so, very positive study. But interestingly, there's one study that shows as you go up, as your vitamin D level goes up too high, let's say you've taken too many vitamin D supplements because you think more is better.

If you have too much vitamin D you may actually increase your risk of colon cancer. As a matter of fact, it increases your risk of cardiovascular disease. That's also something we know, so now we know the range of where we want our vitamin D level to be and that's between 40 to 80 nanomols per litre.

So they concluded that there is a relationship. The lower your vitamin D level is, the higher risk of colon cancer. And also, there's a dose association, so if your vitamin D level goes up 10 nanomols, (vitamin D is measured in the blood as nanomoles per litre [nmol/litre]) your risk goes down 6%, in medical terms, in medicine language that's a huge number and that's good to know.

So how common is vitamin D deficiency? According to the NCHS (U.S. Department of Health) from a study in March of 2011, they determined that 24% of the U.S. population is deficient in vitamin D; that equates to over 1 million persons.

Normal healthy level is 50 to 125 nmol/L, (67% of the population is in this range) risk of deficiency is 30 to 49 nmol/L (24 % of the population is in this range) and the remaining 9%  are < 30 nmol/L.

So this is the national consensus health service data brief. This is the USA 2007 death census, about 2.5 million people died in 2010. Life expectancy is about 78 years. Heart disease is number one, cancer is number two.

## USA 2007 death census
## CDC report 5/2010

| | | | |
|---|---|---|---|
| Number of deaths | 2,423,712 | Heart disease | 616,067 |
| | | Cancer | 562,875 |
| | | Stoke | 135,952 |
| Life expectancy | 77.9 years | Chronic lung disease | 127,924 |
| | | Accidents(unintentional) | 123,706 |
| | | Alzheimer's disease | 74,632 |
| | | Diabetes | 71,382 |
| | | Influenza and Pneumonia | 52,717 |
| | | Nephritis, nephrotic syndrome and nephrosis | 46,448 |
| | | Septicemia | 34,828 |

So how does cancer develop? Apoptosis means cell death. In cancer cells, this doesn't happen, the cancer cells are going to keep dividing and it is not controlled by the body; that is essentially what cancer is, to put it very simple.

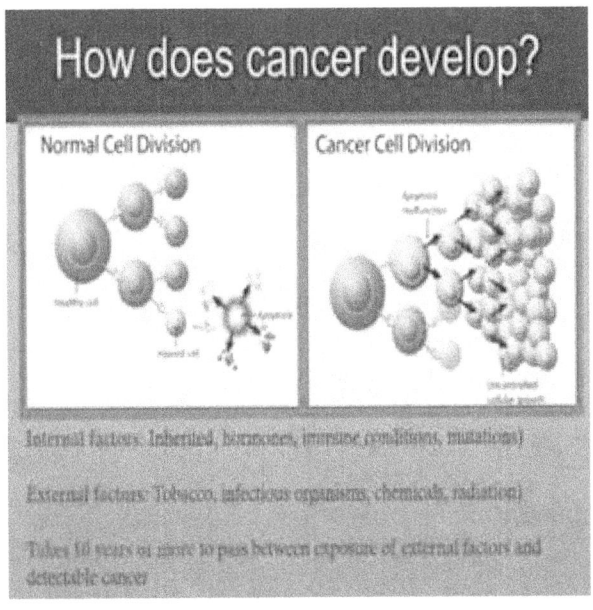

Cancer cells are in a way very smart, they generate their own type of vessels, the more cancer cells you have, the more you will need food. The network of cancer cells grow in a way that is called angiogenesis. They have the ability to produces their own food. Prostate cancer feeds on testosterone. If you block the production of testosterone in the body, the prostate cancer cells will produce its own testosterone. There are many other internal and external factors that contribute to cancer development but they are beyond the scope of this book. Internal factors like hereditary predisposition or external factors like radiation exposure, smoking and so on and so forth.

Let's move forward and look at 25 OH D3 (Vitamin D3), the more potent type of Vitamin D. One way it affects our body is that it triggers the proper absorption of calcium for the bones. You are likely already aware that bone marrow is important for immune system function. Vitamin D is also able to block the proliferation of cancer cells. Not only will it do that, it will also block the cancer cells vessel proliferation. So the actual cancer vessels where cancer is trying to make its own food and grow, vitamin D is going to block that. It prevents both cancer cell division and cancer survival.

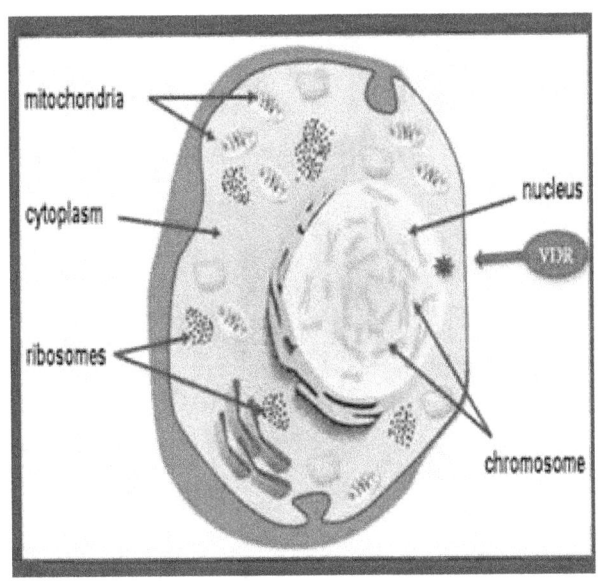

Note the image of the cell above. On each cell, there is what we call a VDR, or a Vitamin D receptor. When you take vitamin D or when your vitamin D levels are normal, this Vitamin D receptor becomes active. When the receptor is active, it will send signals to the chromosomes, (the genes) and these signals are what instruct the cell whether to become cancerous or not.

In this next image you can see that when a cell is damaged, vitamin D is going to be at the source, right when the problem starts, and will give instruction to prevent cancer at the time of cell damage.

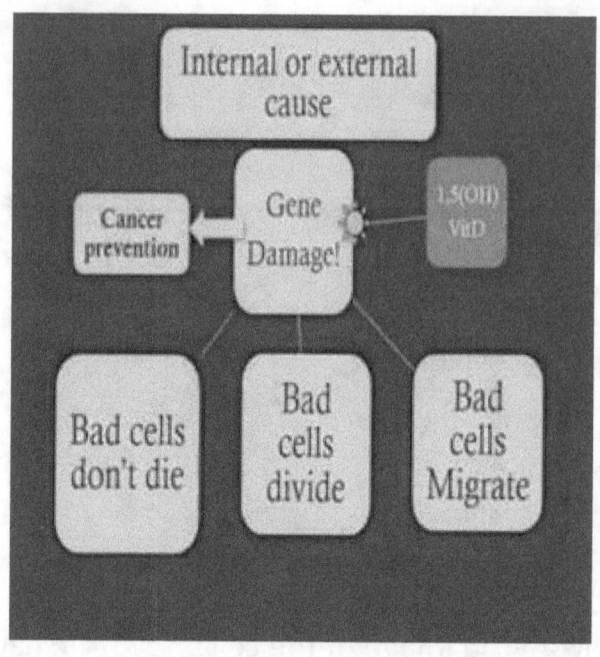

Remember vitamin D receptors are in all cells. Vitamin D actually is a hormone, it is a hormone because it is produced in the body itself. You don't have to have a supplement to have Vitamin D in your body. Hormones affect all the cells and vitamin D is one of them. <u>Low vitamin D does not cause cancer; however low vitamin D levels may prevent the body from having a strong cancer prevention ability at the source of cell damage.</u>

So let's summarize and go over the risk factors that may lead to Vitamin D deficiency. Risk factors in the population include:

- Living in higher latitudes
- Winter season
- Low exposure to the sun
- Dark skinned individuals
- Low absorption ability
- Avid sunscreen users
- Institutionalized individuals
- People who take anti-seizure medication
- Obesity
- People who take steroids or HIV medication
- Pancreatic Insufficiency
- Rare inherited cases
- Vegans

So how much sun exposure do you need to get enough vitamin D? If you exposure a section of your skin, the size of the palm of your hand to the sun on a sunny summer day at noontime for ten minutes; that would be enough to get a healthy daily dose of vitamin D. That is assuming you have a normal level of vitamin D to start with. If you vitamin D is excessively low to start with, you would first have to bring your vitamin D level up to a healthy level before you could apply the above criteria.

Sunscreen does reduce the absorption of UV rays and thus reduces the production of vitamin D, but you will still have some rays get through and you will normally not cover every square inch of your body with sunscreen, for example, the palms of your hands will still be able to absorb the sun's rays for our vitamin D production.

How do you test for vitamin D levels? A blood test will determine your vitamin D level and you can have results quickly, like normally within 3 hours.

Why does obesity negativity affect vitamin D levels?

The reason is because vitamin D is fat soluble and when you have a lot of fat in your body, Vitamin D will be stored in the fat so it will not be available in other areas of the body; it will not be available for your other good cells. This is another good reason to lose weight if you are carrying around excess fat.

Darker skinned individuals get less absorption of Vitamin D from the sun. It would take 1 hour of sun exposure to equal 10 minutes of a fair skinned person.

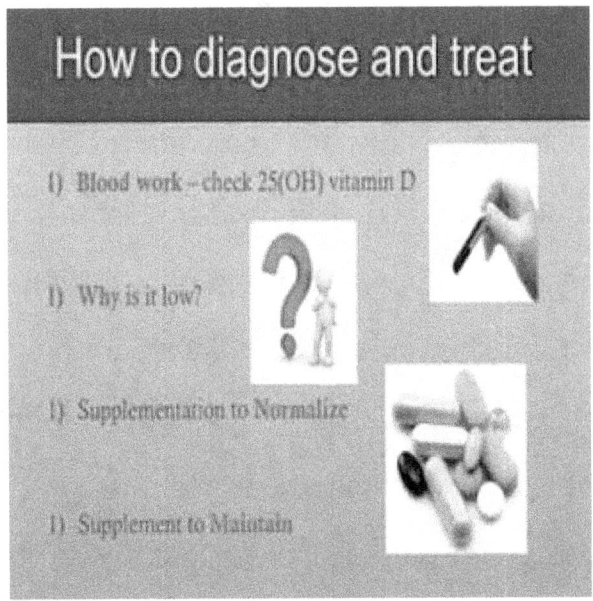

To diagnose vitamin D deficiency, a simple blood test is done. Next they need to determine the cause. It the person has a problem with their digestion, that they cannot digest vitamin D, then there is no point in providing oral supplements. So the doctor will try and normalize the level of vitamin D and then maintain that level.

According to the IOM (Institute of Medicine), a good recommended daily allowance of vitamin D is 600 to 800 IU per day; with a maximum of 4000 IU per day. If a patient that is suffering from vitamin D deficiency and needs to bring the level up, some doctors will start by giving a dose of 50,000 IU once a week for 8 weeks and then measuring the resulting vitamin D level. After this, they will switch to the above daily recommended amounts by the IOM. The IOM is a government agency that gives public recommendations; their recommendations are usually quite conservative.

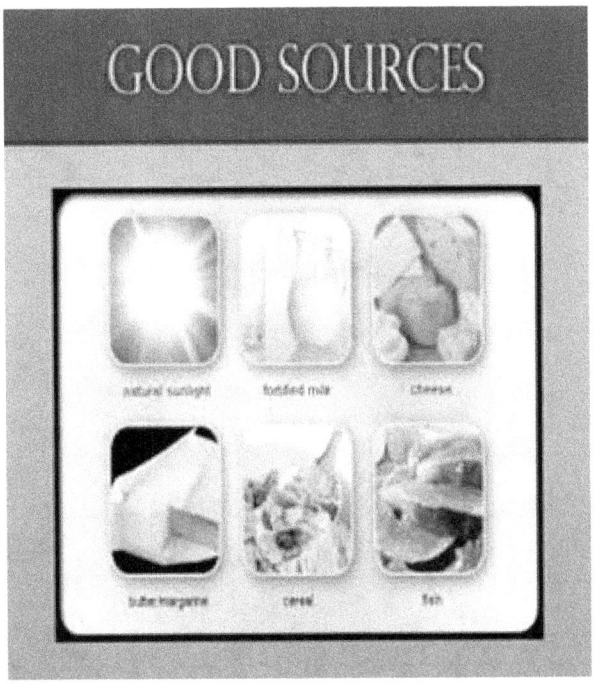

## GOOD SOURCES

natural sunlight — fortified milk — cheese

butter/margarine — cereal — fish

Good sources of vitamin D includes natural sunlight, fortified milk, cheese, butter or margarine, cereal and oily fish like salmon, sardines and mackerel. Although milk is a good source of vitamin D, the type of vitamin D that is added is D2. As we already mentioned, that is not the best type of vitamin D for optimal absorption by the body. The same is true for cheese. Another good source is cod liver oil, which actually provides the highest concentration of vitamin D per ounce. (1360 IU per ounce).

## Food sources

| Food | Serving Size | Vitamin D (IU) |
|---|---|---|
| Pink Salmon, canned | 3 ounces | 530 |
| Sardines, canned | 3 ounces | 231 |
| Tuna, Canned | 3 ounces | 200 |
| Cow's milk | 8 ounces | 100 |
| Orange juice fortified with Vitamin D | 8 ounces | 100 |
| Fortified Breakfast cereal | 1 serving (1 cup) | 40-50 |
| Egg | 1 ounce | 20 |
| Cod liver oil | 1 ounce | 1,360 |

If a person is a vegan, they may want to stick with taking Vitamin D2 since that is produced from plant sources. In fact Vitamin D2 will often be labeled as vegan. If maintaining a vegan diet is not important, then D3 is the way to go. You can see from the image below that the chemical composition is very similar with D3 just having one extra methyl group in the makeup.

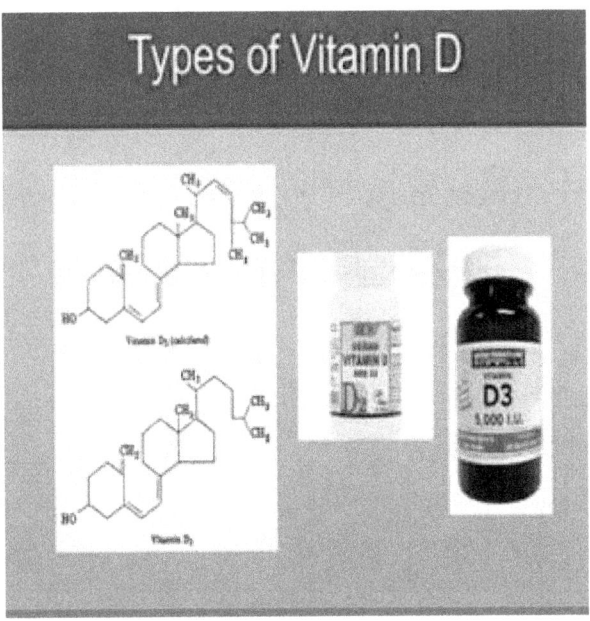

*Vitamin D2 and D3 very similar in chemical composition.*

So to conclude this important section on Vitamin D and cancer, remember these points:

Vitamin D deficiency is common.

Vitamin D affects many organs.

Cancer risk goes up with low Vitamin D levels. This is true for any type of cancer.

Ask a doctor to check your vitamin D levels with a simple blood test. Twice a year is a good idea.

Try to get most of your vitamin D from good food sources but don't neglect supplementation.

## Vitamin D and Psoriasis

Researcher Michael Holick came up with the idea of wondering whether Vitamin D would help the skin itself. Since the skin had the design for making use of Vitamin from sunlight, he reasoned that there must be a direct benefit to the skin itself from having exposure to the suns UV rays and using it to create Vitamin D. So he created a topical treatment by combing Vitamin D3 with Vaseline to create a simple method of application.

He then contacted dermatologists who sent him a patient suffering from psoriasis on his arms for eight years and who had never responded favorably to any other treatment. Here is an image of his arms before treatment:

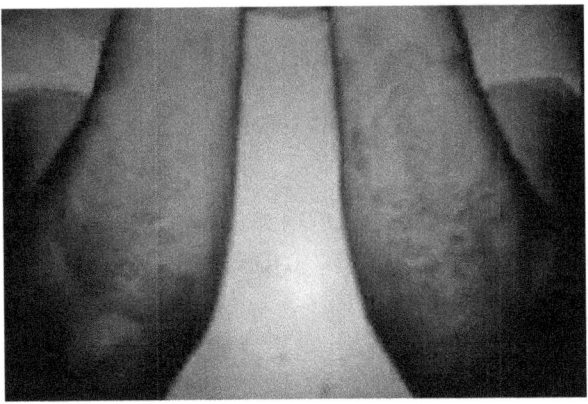

Then he started using two tubes of the prepared Vitamin D3 ointment. On one side he used one tube and on the other side, he used the other tube. One of the tubes contained the prepared Vitamin D3 application and the other tube contained no Vitamin D3; it was just a placebo in the second tube. Neither the doctor nor the patient knew which tube was which.

After 3 months, the patient returned and showed the results in the following image:

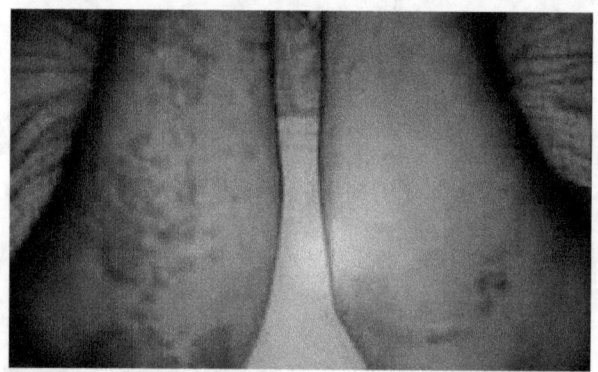

You can see that the results are dramatic. The left side was the placebo and the right side was the result with the vitamin D3 application.

Here is another example of an individual suffering from scalp psoriasis:

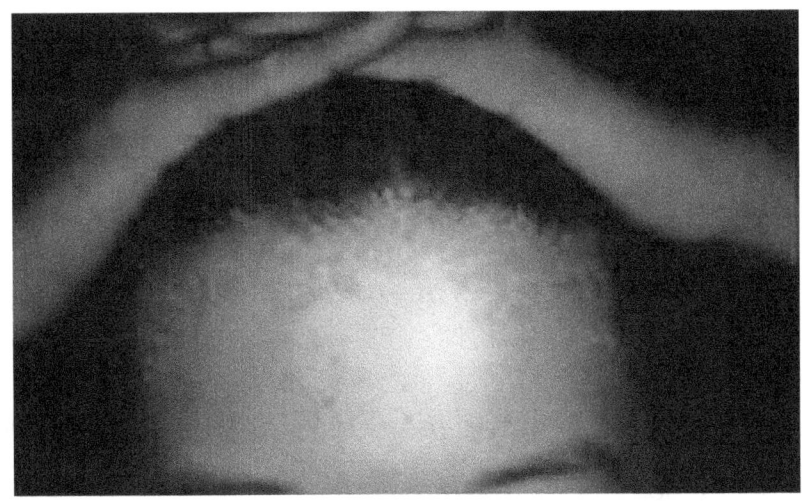

And here is the picture after being treated with a topical treatment of Vitamin D3:

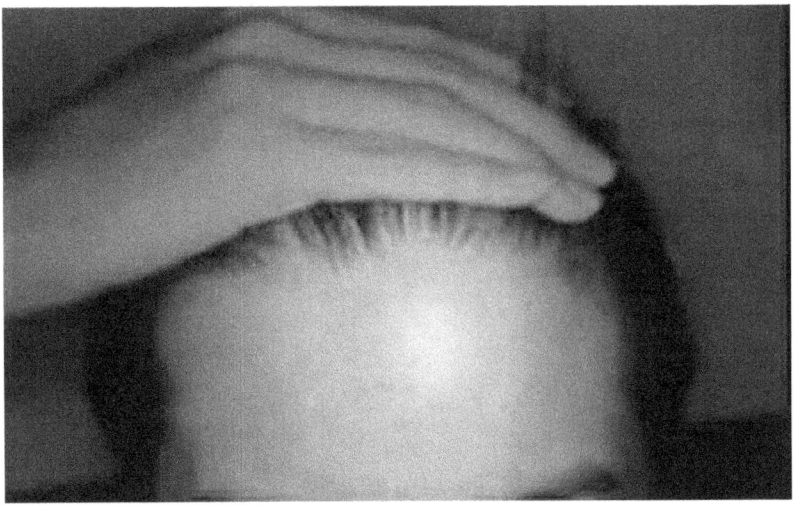

Once again, you can see that the results are dramatic.

## Suggested Vitamin D Retail Products

At once time, you would never find Vitamin D stocked in pharmacies but now of course, it is readily available.

On a recent trip to my local pharmacy I found the following to choose from:

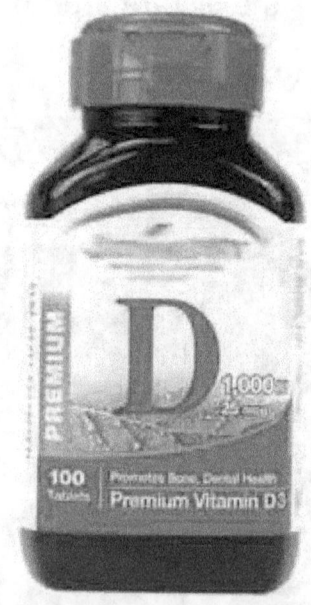

This particular brand (I've blurred out the brand name) was selling for $12.98 for 100 tablets. Each tablet contained 1000 IU of Vitamin D3. The saleslady mentioned that they sometimes had them on a BOGO sale (Buy one, get one free). If they were on sale then the effective price would be half or $6.49 per bottle.

I also found this other brand:

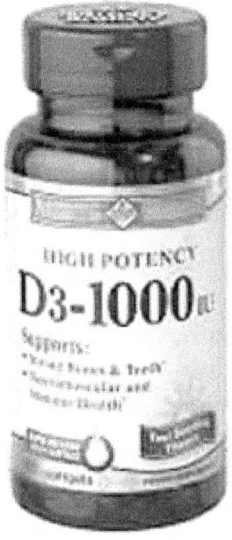

This brand was providing 120 tablets that each also contained 1000 IU of Vitamin D3. They were available as chewable mixed berry flavor tablets for a price of only $5.99 so this was clearly the better deal providing twenty percent more product at a lower price and in a nice tasting format!

As you can see, the cost of Vitamin D3 is very reasonable and the low cost makes it even more compelling to make sure that supplementation is a part of your diet. Be sure to compare prices and brands as the prices can fluctuate a lot as seen in the examples above.

Sometimes Vitamin D tablets are sold together with Calcium. Since Vitamin D regulates Calcium metabolism, it makes sense to take these two together. If you are getting sufficient calcium in your diet already, simply taking Vitamin D alone will help your body use the Calcium that your diet already provides.

## Summary and Conclusion

The current research shows that Vitamin D deficiency is common widespread especially in individuals that get limited sun exposure. We now know that Vitamin D affects many, if not all, of the organs in our body and in fact every cell has a VDR – a Vitamin D Receptor that is able to send signals to the chromosomes. These signals include instructions about cell replication and overall cell health. Consequently cancer risk goes up with low Vitamin D levels. Low vitamin D levels may be a contributing factor in the progression for any type of cancer.

Ask a doctor to check your vitamin D levels with a simple blood test. Twice a year is a good idea. You want to make sure that your vitamin D level in your blood is at least 50 nanomoles per litre. If it is below this level, you can take large doses of vitamin D to get your level back to normal. For example you could take 50,000 IU once a week for 8 weeks. Then maintain a healthy level by taking 1000 IU of Vitamin D3 once a day.

Try to get most of your vitamin D from good food sources but don't neglect supplementation. And lastly and most importantly, take control of your own health!

# Appendix 1

From the NCBI, (National Center for Biotechnology Information)

## Osteoporosis: Can calcium and vitamin D prevent it?

Older people can reduce their risk of osteoporosis by taking calcium supplements every day. It is not clear whether extra **vitamin D** helps to strengthen people's bones if they do not have a vitamin D deficiency.

Osteoporosis is when bones become weaker and brittle because of a loss of bone tissue. Bones affected by osteoporosis are much more likely to break. Even a minor fall could cause a break or crack in the bone (fracture). Osteoporosis is common in people over the age of 65, but the risk of developing osteoporosis starts increasing from around the age of 50. For women, the risk of osteoporosis also increases quite a lot after menopause.

Sometimes there are obvious signs that a person has osteoporosis – they may lose some height and stoop over, for example. But often the first sign that someone has developed osteoporosis is when they break a bone.

One of the main building blocks of bone is the mineral called calcium. Normal healthy bones turn over calcium constantly. Calcium in our diets is absorbed by our bones and released again, with new calcium coming in to offset the loss. One of the factors weakening the bones of people with osteoporosis is that their bones are losing far too much calcium. So one possible approach to preventing osteoporosis is to increase the amount of calcium they consume, either with a calcium-rich diet or with the help of dietary supplements. Calcium supplements are available without prescription, either as calcium alone or combined with vitamin D.

Vitamin D helps bones absorb calcium. Many people who are very old have a vitamin D deficiency, partly because they are no longer so active, leave the house less often, and get too little sunlight. Our bodies can make their own vitamin D if we get enough sunlight. But there is also vitamin D in some foods, so that we can also get vitamin D in our diets or through dietary supplements.

**The results of trials in close to 64,000 people over the age of 50.**

Researchers from three universities in Australia worked together to find out whether dietary supplements can really prevent osteoporosis and, if so, how much supplementation is needed. They looked for trials that had tested what happens when people over the age of 50 take calcium supplements, with or without vitamin D, to try to prevent osteoporosis. The trials had to have found out how many people went on to have fractures, or at least measured the participants' bone-mineral density.

The researchers found 29 trials where almost 64,000 people had agreed to be randomly placed in one of two groups: in one they received real supplements, and in the other fake supplements (placebos). The research volunteers in these randomized controlled trials were not told which group they were in. So they did not know whether they were given the tablets with calcium or the ones without it. Whatever differences there were in their bones at the end of the trial are therefore very likely to be caused by the differences in the tablets they were taking. In other types of scientific research people who volunteer to take real supplements might be more motivated and health-conscious than average. This could influence the results of the research.

The people in the trials were nearly all women. In fact, 92% of the participants were women. But because so many people participated, there were still thousands of men in the trials: enough for the researchers to be able to show that the results were much the same for men as for women.

The results were clear. People who take these dietary supplements are less likely to lose bone density, and their bones are a little less likely to break. The risk is already reduced within only 3.5 years of taking the supplements, as long as they are taken regularly.

### A lower risk of fractured bones.

Most of the people who were taking real supplements in the trials had tablets to take every day that contained at least 1,000 mg of calcium. However, not everyone took the tablets very regularly. But even including all the participants who did not take the tablets regularly, there was a small overall reduction in fractures. The number of fractures was researched in over 52,000 participants.

People who took real calcium supplements were less likely to fracture their bones. This effect was particularly clear in those over the age of 70 who took the tablets very regularly: an extra 1 out of 30 were spared any broken bones. In younger people this protective effect was smaller, so it is not clear how much they benefit from taking calcium supplements over long periods of time.

The researchers came to the following conclusions:

- A dose of 1,000 to 1,200 mg calcium a day is probably necessary to reduce the risk of fracture, especially if a person's diet is low in calcium.

- Adding up to 800 IU of vitamin D to the calcium probably makes no difference. (IU = international units; an internationally defined measurement for the amount of a substance). It is not clear if higher doses of vitamin D will improve the results.

- People at higher risk of fractures benefit more from taking calcium supplements. That includes people who are much older than 50, people who have a lower body weight, those who have less calcium in their diets, or people who are living in institutions.

- People who take calcium supplements have higher bone density in their hips and spines.

- Both women and men benefit from calcium supplementation.

## How much is too much?

This research did not look at the issues of safety and adverse effects from dietary supplements. The level of 1,000 to 1,300 mg is about the recommended daily level of intake for calcium in Europe and the U.S. But, of course, the calcium taken in a supplement is additional to the calcium that people are getting in their diets. The people in these trials had varying amounts of calcium in their diets. European authorities recommend that adults do not have more than a total of 2,500 to 3,000 mg of calcium a day from all sources. The German Federal Institute for Risk Assessment recommends people aged 65 or older not to take more vitamin D supplements than 400 IU per day.

Some researchers have found a possible risk of heart attack when people who already take in more than 800 mg of calcium a day in their diet also use calcium supplements. Combining calcium supplements with vitamin D might lower this effect.

One of the trials included in this research is the big American Women's Health Initiative trial in women after menopause. More than 18,000 women were in the group given daily supplements with 1,000 mg of calcium plus 400 IU of vitamin D. One adverse effect that the researchers identified was a small increase in kidney stones. Compared to the women taking placebos, that happened to about 4 more women out of every 1,000 women who took the supplements. But the women who developed kidney stones were not necessarily those who had particularly high levels of calcium in their diets.

Researchers from the U.S. government Agency for Health Care Quality and Research concluded that the development of kidney stones is the only relevant side effect that has been identified in trials. However, the World Health Organization (WHO) has identified kidney stones as a possible side effect of high vitamin D intake. If you are concerned about your risk of kidney stones, make sure you drink water regularly. This can help lower that risk.

Researchers are also still studying whether or not calcium supplements might be able to prevent bowel cancer.

# Appendix 2

From the NCBI, (National Center for Biotechnology Information)

**Rickets**, the clinical disorder of vitamin D deficiency during infancy and childhood, is deemed a relic of the past by modern-day clinicians in the United States. However, this apparently vanquished nutritional or sunlight-deprivation disorder is making a comeback. Recent case reports highlight the resurgence of rickets among infants who had been exclusively breastfed beyond 6 months of age without vitamin D supplementation. The majority of the affected infants were dark skinned (Black, Afro-Caribbean, or of Asian descent), residents of northern latitudes, or both.

## Breastfeeding and the Emergence of Rickets

Maternal vitamin D status is an important factor for the development of rickets in breastfed infants. Typically, breast-milk lacks adequate vitamin D unless the nursing mother is adequately supplemented with vitamin D or exposed to enough sunlight. Humans meet their vitamin D needs from sunlight exposure and diet; however, very few foods are naturally rich in vitamin D.

The vitamin D precursor (7-dehydrocholesterol) in the skin is photolyzed into previtamin $D_3$ upon exposure to a narrow band of solar ultraviolet-B (UV-B) photons (290–315 nm). Previtamin $D_3$ is rapidly converted to vitamin $D_3$, which is further hydroxylated in the liver to 25-hydroxyvitamin $D_3$ [25(OH)$D_3$] and then in the kidney to 1,25-dihydroxyvitamin $D_3$, the active form of vitamin $D_3$. 25(OH)D is the major circulating vitamin D metabolite, and its measure reflects the vitamin D status of an individual.

Vitamin $D_3$ photoproduction is influenced by season, latitude of residence, and skin color. Wintertime vitamin $D_3$ photoproduction is compromised in latitudes above 35°. During winter in the higher latitudes, sunlight has a longer tangential path to reach the earth's surface, resulting in the absorption and loss of the UV-B photons in the ozone stratosphere. The role of skin color in vitamin $D_3$ photoproduction hinges on the function of melanin. Epidermal melanin concentration determines an individual's skin color, and dark-skinned individuals have higher levels of cutaneous melanin.

The vitamin $D_3$ precursor, 7-dehydrocholesterol, is predominantly concentrated in the viable deeper layers of the epidermis, namely the stratum spinosum and stratum basale. Melanin acts as a natural filter (sunscreen) and efficiently absorbs the UV-B photons, compromising vitamin $D_3$ photoproduction in dark-skinned people. These individuals need upwards of 6-times greater exposure to UV-B radiation to raise their vitamin $D_3$ levels to the same level as in White individuals. Dark-skinned people residing in the northeastern United States are vulnerable year-round—but especially in the winter—to hypovitaminosis D (i.e., vitamin D insufficiency) because of their skin color and inadequate sunlight exposure.

It is apparent that the current reemergence of rickets has coincided with a resurgence of breast-feeding without adequate vitamin D supplementation. The prevalence of hypovitaminosis D is particularly marked among Black women, 42% of whom in the reproductive age group (age 15–49 years) have the condition.

Data from the National Health and Nutrition Examination Survey (NHANES) 1999–2000 showed that non-Hispanic Blacks had consistently lower intakes of vitamin D from food and supplements than did Whites. It is therefore not surprising that we are seeing cases of rickets among breastfed dark-skinned infants. Currently, however, there are no guidelines for optimizing and monitoring the vitamin D status of dark-skinned nursing mothers.

Recognizing that prolonged breastfeeding without adequate vitamin D supplementation is an important risk factor for rickets, the American Academy of Pediatrics in April 2003 recommended that all breastfed infants, irrespective of skin color or latitude of residence, be given 200 IU of vitamin D per day. This recommendation, however, is still inadequate for addressing the problem of reemerging rickets. **The Canadian Government has mandated that all breastfed infants receive 400 IU of vitamin D daily.**

The reemergence of rickets could also be ascribed to the avoidance of direct exposure to sunlight among infants less than 6 months of age, as a preventive measure for reducing the risk of skin cancer during adulthood associated with early exposure to ultraviolet radiation from sunlight. Even though overt vitamin D deficiency and rickets remain uncommon in the United States, hypovitaminosis D, characterized by low levels of 25(OH)D (< 20 ng/mL), is thought to be more pervasive. Epidemiological and clinical studies have highlighted the excessive prevalence of hypovitaminosis D among apparently healthy children, adolescents, and adults worldwide. In this context, we reviewed the history of rickets, focusing on the discovery of vitamin D, a seminal event in public health's conquest of the rickets epidemic of the early 20th century.

## History of Rickets

Rickets, being a sun-deprivation disorder, most likely affected early residents of the world's temperate climates. Soranus of Ephesus, a famous physician of the Greco-Roman Era (1st–2nd century AD), observed bony deformities suggestive of rickets among infants residing in Rome. It was not until the mid-17th century, however, that rickets was readily recognized as a distinct disease. By then, rickets was endemic among residents of the southwest counties of Dorset and Somerset in England. The mid-17th-century "endemic" of rickets could be explained by this population's urbanization. The concomitant atmospheric pollution resulting in smoke and smog would have hindered the sun-mediated vitamin D synthesis in the population and increased their vulnerability for rickets.

The first published account of rickets as a clinical disease is credited to Daniel Whistler in 1645. Whistler wrote his monograph *Inaugural Medical Disputation on the Disease of English Children Which Is Popularly Termed the Rickets*, a concise description of clinical features and symptoms of rickets, as a thesis for his doctor of medicine degree in October 1645 from Leyden, in the Netherlands. Whistler's work, however, was soon eclipsed by Francis Glisson's treatise on rickets, *De Rachitide*, or *On Rickets*, published in 1650.

Unlike Whistler, Glisson described rickets on the basis of clinical and postmortem experience with the condition. Glisson's work, which remains a classic, should be credited with highlighting the importance of morbid anatomy in the description of a clinical disorder.

Little progress in the understanding of rickets was made for the next two and a half centuries. At the dawn of the 20th century, the expansive industrialization and urban migration in the major cities of western Europe and the northern United States set the stage for the high prevalence of rickets among infants residing in those polluted and "sunless" cities. Overcrowded living conditions in the big-city slums and tenements and the sunlight deprivation precipitated by atmospheric pollution from smoke and smog were responsible for a rickets epidemic. Increased ozone concentration from industrial pollution and the haze and clouds from atmospheric pollution compromise vitamin D production by absorbing the UV-B photons essential for its synthesis.

The first two and a half decades of the 20th century saw phenomenal advances in the understanding of rickets: the induction of experimental rickets in animal models and the understanding of histological changes in rickets, the delineation of the anti-rachitic properties of cod liver oil and ultraviolet irradiation, and the use of biochemical and radiological tests in the study of rickets.

Alfred F. Hess, a New York pediatrician and pioneering nutritional researcher in the early 20th century, fondly referred to this period as the "second great chapter" in the history of rickets and its renaissance period.

The medical benefits of cod liver oil, although not as a specific anti-rachitic agent, were recognized in the folklore of the coastal residents of northern Europe. Use of cod liver oil specifically to prevent rickets was first reported by D. Schutte in 1824,and German and French physicians recommended cod liver oil for this purpose during the rest of the century. Unfortunately, during the rickets epidemic in Europe and the northern United States at the turn of the 20th century, the specific anti-rachitic properties of cod liver oil were not universally acknowledged and the medical establishment had become skeptical about its usefulness, perhaps because prescribed cod liver oil was often of poor quality or contained impurities.

Classic animal experiments by Edward Mellanby and Elmer McCollum established irrevocably the anti-rachitic properties of cod liver oil. They ascribed the anti-rachitic function of cod liver oil to "fat soluble A" (or vitamin A, which is present in high concentrations in cod liver oil) or a similar substance.

In 1922, McCollum demonstrated that heated cod liver oil lost its protectiveness against vitamin A deficiency (dryness of the conjunctiva and cornea [xerophthalmia] and softening of the cornea [keratomalacia]) but still retained its anti-rachitic function. He coined the term "vitamin D" to refer to the anti-rachitic factor in cod liver oil, as it was fourth in the sequence of vitamins discovered.

As faith in cod liver oil as an anti-rachitic agent was being restored, the role of ultraviolet radiation as a therapeutic agent in rickets was established. In 1919, Kurt Huldschinsky cured rickets in infants by exposing them to light rays from a mercury vapor lamp. As early as 1822, Jedrzej Sniadecki, a Polish physician, had observed that rates of rickets were higher among infants residing in the polluted, sunless tenements of the inner-city areas of Warsaw than in rural areas; he identified lack of exposure to sunlight as the etiologic factor for rickets.

In 1890, Theobald Palm observed the negative relationship between latitude and occurrence of rickets. In the sunny tropics, despite poverty and poor sanitation, rickets among infants was rarer than in temperate climates, where living conditions and diet were better. Palm recognized the benefits of sunlight in the prevention and treatment of rickets and recommended the "systematic use of sun-baths as a preventive and therapeutic measure in rickets." He also suggested that infants and children afflicted with rickets be moved "as early as possible from large towns to a locality where sunshine abounds and the air is dry and bracing."

Establishment of the fact that cod liver oil and sunlight were distinct but similar in their ability to prevent and treat rickets was a significant advance in the study of rickets during the early 20th century.

In 1923, Martha May Eliot, a faculty pediatrician at Yale School of Medicine and a member of the United States Children's Bureau, began a pioneering 3-year communitywide demonstration project in New Haven, Conn, to explore the efficacy of cod liver oil and sunlight in the prevention of rickets. Infants born in the study district during the first 2 years of the study were enrolled and underwent monthly clinical and radiological assessments for rickets. Eliot showed that prophylactic cod liver oil and sunlight therapy were effective in preventing or reversing the disease's progression. This discovery led to a public health campaign for sensible sun exposure and food fortification with vitamin $D_2$, a major step in the eradication of the rickets epidemic. Vitamin $D_2$ (ergocalciferol) is derived from ultraviolet radiation of ergosterol, a vitamin D precursor naturally found in yeast and fungi (ergot) and was the first photosynthesized vitamin D used for food fortification.

**Sunlight and Rickets**

The medical benefits of sunlight were recognized as early as 1822 by Sniadecki. In 1903, Auguste Rollier established a natural heliotherapy center at Leysin in the Swiss Alps to treat patients with symptomatic tuberculosis by exposure to sunlight. Rollier empirically recognized the benefit of heliotherapy for the cure of rickets as early as 1916. In his book on heliotherapy published in 1923, he acknowledged Huldschinsky's discovery of curing rickets with ultraviolet rays as "the beginnings of a scientific foundation for our own purely empirical conclusions. Sun and ultraviolet rays bear much the same relation to one another as crude drugs do to their synthetically prepared chemical substitutes."

Hess had critically appraised the seasonal variation in the occurrence of rickets among his pediatric patients in the context of their diet. In 1922, as a practicing pediatrician in New York City, he was aware that rickets was most prevalent among his patients at the end of March, when it was present in nearly 50% of the breastfed infants despite adequate maternal nutrition.

Hess noted that "breast-milk, although valuable, is provided with but a scant factor of safety against rickets, and . . . additional protective influence is needed— namely, light." As Sniadecki had done 100 years earlier, Hess identified lack of sunlight as the dominant etiologic agent in the rickets epidemic observed in temperate climates since the time of Glisson.

In the development of experimental or clinical rickets, sunlight has a reciprocal relationship to diet, rate of growth, and the degree of skin pigmentation. Animals protected from rickets by exposure to a constant dose of sunlight become vulnerable to rickets if their rate of growth increases, because rickets is a metabolic state of defective mineralization of the growing bones. Compared with a normally growing infant, an infant with growth failure is relatively protected against rickets and may need less sunlight to stave it off. The degree of skin pigmentation determines the efficacy of sunlight. In 1917, Hess and Lester Unger observed rickets in nearly 90% of

Black infants residing in the Columbus Hill District, a Black neighborhood in New York City.

Race, diet, rate of growth, geographic latitude of residence, customs, religion, culture, and environmental pollution are factors that modify the influence of sunlight on rickets. Religion and culture play a role in the development of rickets and vitamin D deficiency among breastfed infants from sunny locales such as the Middle East or first-generation infants from Middle Eastern immigrant families residing in North America, Europe, or Australia. The custom of wearing traditional clothing that covers most of the body leads to sunlight deprivation in the mother and clinical or subclinical vitamin D deficiency in the nursing infant.

Hess and several other investigators were able to establish that mere exposure to sunlight could cure rickets. Establishing the chemical basis of heliotherapy in the treatment of rickets was the next step. John Howland and Benjamin Kramer observed consistently low serum phosphorus levels in infants with active rickets and noted that cod liver oil therapy cured the rickets and normalized the serum phosphorus. Hess and Margaret Gutman observed the impact of direct sunlight on rickets and phosphorus levels in a cohort of 7 infants (aged 7 to 37 months) from June through September 1921. They found that sunlight therapy improved the clinical and radiological status of rickets and increased mean phosphorus levels from 3.11 mg/dL (low) to 4.02 mg/dL (normal). Hess and Gutman thus established the chemical basis of heliotherapy and showed that the curative processes of sunlight and cod liver oil therapy were similar. They claimed that their results "furnish the first definitive evidence of metabolic change in the animal body brought about by the solar rays."

### Ultraviolet Radiation and Rickets

Understanding that the anti-rachitic potency of sunlight and artificial light was limited to a narrow band of ultraviolet radiation was the next major advance in the history of vitamin $D_3$. Hess showed that exposure to a mercury vapor lamp (spectral range=230–595 nm) for 3 minutes from a distance of 3 feet prevented the onset of rickets in rats maintained on a standard diet. Interposing a Corning window glass filter (2.6mm thickness) rendered the mercury vapor lamplight ineffective at preventing rickets. The filter blocked ultraviolet rays of less than 334 nm, suggesting that these wavelengths were responsible for the anti-rachitic effect.

Hess and Mildred Weinstock further characterized the anti-rachitic spectra of ultraviolet radiation. They studied the prevention of rickets in 4-week-old rats on a rachitogenic diet by exposing them to various spectra and intensities of ultraviolet radiation generated from a mercury vapor lamp with special filters. The animals were X-rayed after 21 days and were screened for the histological presence of rickets after 28 days. They concluded that the spectra of ultraviolet rays protective against rickets "have a wave length not longer than 302 or possibly 313 millimicrons [nanometers]."

## Prevention of Rickets by Filtered Mecury Vapor Lamp Rays

Ultraviolet radiation from the sun constitutes less than 1% of total solar radiation, and the shortest waves of sunlight reaching the surface of the earth are 290 nm. It is therefore only a narrow band of the sun's ultraviolet radiation (290–315 nm) that influences the vitamin $D_3$ status, bone health, and calcium economy of humans. According to Hess, the quantity and quality of the anti-rachitic ultraviolet spectrum of sunlight is "circumscribed by nature and furthermore limited by natural and artificial meteorological conditions." Seasonal variation in the anti-rachitic ultraviolet spectrum of sunlight was the dominant factor in the excessive prevalence of rickets during winter among infants residing in the temperate climes during the early part of the 20th century. Variation in the ultraviolet spectrum of sunlight reaching the earth's surface hinges on altitude and latitude, season of the year, time of day, and atmospheric pollution; however, Hess wrote, "the dominant factor in regard to the anti-rachitic activity of solar rays is not so much the number of hours of sunshine as its quality and intensity."

### Activation of Vitamin D in Foods by Ultraviolet Radiation

The quest to trap the sun's radiant energy in foods to render them anti-rachitic soon followed. The role of sunlight in rickets was shrouded in mystery. It was evident that direct ultraviolet irradiation could promote growth in rats maintained on a vitamin D–deficient diet containing a high calcium and low phosphorus content. Ultraviolet irradiation from mercury vapor lamps promoted growth in rats failing to thrive on diets deficient in fat-soluble vitamin A, despite the rats' overt vitamin A deficiency (progressive xerophthalmia). Heated and oxidized cod liver oil (devoid of vitamin A) was comparable to ultraviolet irradiation in growth promotion, suggesting that the anti-rachitic agent in ultraviolet radiation and cod liver oil were identical in function.

In 1923, Eleanor Hume and Hannah Smith reported from England that rats transferred to "empty" jars that were previously exposed to ultraviolet radiation grew as well as rats that were irradiated directly; they concluded that "irradiated air" was imparted with a growth-promoting property. Attempts to corroborate their study, however, were unsuccessful.

E.M. Nelson and Harry Steenbock of the University of Wisconsin at Madison were aware of Hume and Smith's report and speculated that the protection noted in the "empty" irradiated jars was perhaps because of the activation of residual sawdust or foods that were not removed prior to the irradiation of the jars. They were intrigued by the results of their own irradiation experiments. Much to their amazement, rats maintained on a rachitogenic diet began to grow when irradiated rats were introduced into their cage. They attributed the growth promotion in the nonirradiated rats to the ingestion of the "photochemically activated" excreta of the irradiated rats.

Steenbock and Archie Black irradiated foods to see if they could be rendered anti-rachitic. They presumed that foods that caused growth failure in rats that did not show signs of overt vitamin A deficiency were deficient in the anti-rachitic factor. When they exposed such foods to a mercury vapor lamp and fed them to rachitic rats, the foods promoted growth and calcium assimilation in the rats, similar to what happened when the rats were irradiated directly. Steenbock realized the potential of his discovery and chose to patent it to prevent the misuse of the irradiation process and to monitor the advertisements, claims, and quality of irradiated products.

Soon after Steenbock published his findings, Hess and Weinstock reported similar results. Cottonseed oil, linseed oil, wheat germ, and lettuce deemed inert and ineffective for treating rickets were made potent anti-rachitic agents by ultraviolet irradiation. They speculated that if the anti-rachitic factor in the irradiated foods was similar to cod liver oil, it should be considered a vitamin, and their results would "constitute the first demonstration of the production of vitamin in vitro." Hess did not foresee the commercial potential for activation of foods by ultraviolet irradiation and suggested that "the therapeutic value of this procedure is of secondary importance" and perhaps of value only in the event of cod liver oil shortage.

The discovery that ultraviolet irradiation of foods could render them anti-rachitic was a major breakthrough. It became possible to enhance the vitamin D content of common infant foods such as milk and cereal in an inexpensive and palatable way. Consumption of such vitamin D–enhanced foods led to the eradication of "epidemic" rickets. People were advised to take their "daily dose of sunshine" in their diet. Within 2 decades, a wide variety of foods and beverages were fortified with vitamin D, including bread, custard, soda, hot dogs, and even beer.

## Steenbock Patents

Steenbock wanted to patent his irradiation process to ensure the quality of the commercially produced vitamin D–enhanced irradiated foods and to protect the Wisconsin dairy industry from the oleomargarine industry. Unlike butter, margarine, a cheap butter substitute, lacked vitamins A and D; however, margarine could be fortified with vitamin A. Steenbock was convinced that the Wisconsin dairy industry would suffer if the oleomargarine manufacturers had access to a process for vitamin D enrichment.

Steenbock asked the University of Wisconsin to manage his patents. The response from the Board of Regents was tentative and lukewarm, as there was no precedence for patent management. Realizing the prospects of Steenbock's discovery, Harry L. Russell, dean of the College of Agriculture, and Charles S. Slichter, dean of the Graduate School, convinced several alumni to create an independent organization to handle the patents. Thus, the Wisconsin Alumni Research Foundation (WARF) was founded on November 14, 1925, to administer Steenbock's patents. WARF granted the licenses for using the irradiation process and functioned as an intermediary between the university and commerce. It ensured the quality of irradiated products and monitored the appropriateness of the manufacturers' advertising claims. WARF was able to deny licensing to the oleo-margarine industry, thereby ensuring the commercial viability of Wisconsin's dairy industry, the driving force of the state's agricultural economy. The monies generated from the licenses were used exclusively for the promotion of research at the University of Wisconsin.

Quaker Oats received the first license from WARF in February 1927 to manufacture vitamin D–enriched breakfast cereal. Licenses were issued to pharmaceutical companies (Abbott Laboratories, Mead Johnson, Parke

Davis, Winthrop Chemical Co, and Squibb) to manufacture a medicinal vitamin D product called Viosterol (irradiated ergosterol). By 1934, the irradiation process was extended to produce vitamin D–fortified milk. Soon, vitamin D fortification was achieved inexpensively by adding vitamin D directly to milk. The advent and consumption of vitamin D–fortified foods led to the eradication of rickets. Vitamin D food fortification was a public health triumph. Photosynthesis of vitamin D in foods by ultraviolet irradiation, made feasible by the seminal discoveries of Steenbock and Hess, was instrumental in this success.

### The Nature of Sunshine Vitamin D

The chemical nature of vitamin D was yet to be discerned. The vitamin D precursor substrate, activated by irradiation, was traced to the "sterol" fraction of foods, phytosterol in vegetable foods and to cholesterol in animal foods. Hess et al. demonstrated that phytosterol obtained from cottonseed oil and cholesterol obtained from brain tissue could be rendered anti-rachitic by ultraviolet irradiation. With intuition, they hypothesized that ultraviolet irradiation from solar rays and artificial sources activates the cholesterol in the skin to render it anti-rachitic and suggested that the proposed mechanism "presupposes not only formation of active cholesterol within the skin but its further transport by way of circulation." Huldschinsky showed that irradiation of 1 arm could cure the rickets in the other, suggesting that something made in the skin had to enter the circulation to impart the cure.

Chemical purification of the sterols was attempted to help further delineate the exact nature of the vitamin D precursor. It was realized that the vitamin D precursor in cholesterol rendered anti-rachitic by ultraviolet irradiation was a contaminant and not a part of the purified cholesterol. An international collaborative effort between Hess (New York, NY), Adolf Windaus (Gottingen, Germany), and Otto Rosenheim (London, England) was responsible for identifying and clarifying the nature of the vitamin D precursor "contaminant" in cholesterol. Spectroscopic absorption studies highlighted that the vitamin D precursor fraction of cholesterol exhibited 3 absorption peaks (269, 280, 293 nm). From these data, they identified the vitamin D precursor fraction as ergosterol, which is typically found in yeast and fungi (ergot). Irradiated ergosterol (also known as ergocalciferol, calciferol, viosterol, and vitamin $D_2$) was the first photosynthesized anti-rachitic agent to be discovered.

The vitamin D precursor factor in animals or humans that, through exposure to ultraviolet irradiation, became anti-rachitic had to be different because ergosterol is distributed only in plants and fungi. In 1934, J. Waddell demonstrated that the vitamin D precursor in cod liver oil and irradiated nonpurified cholesterol was different from ergosterol. Windaus and F. Bock identified the vitamin D precursor in animal skin as 7-dehydrocholesterol. Irradiated 7-dehydrocholesterol was the photosynthesized anti-rachitic agent in the skin and in foods of animal origin; it came to be called vitamin $D_3$, or cholecalciferol.


## Conclusion

We have reviewed the story of the discovery of photosynthesized vitamin D. Edwards Park states, "But for rickets vitamin D would not have been discovered. Its discovery was the secret to rickets; its use is essentially the therapy of that disease." The discovery of vitamin D led to the eradication of the epidemic rickets of the early 20th century. Pioneering advances were made in the understanding of vitamin D and rickets from 1915 to 1935. The discovery of the synthesis of vitamin D by the irradiation of foods was the "jewel in the crown" of vitamin D discoveries. This discovery was a catalyst for the public health triumph against rickets. It became feasible to fortify and enrich milk and other foods with vitamin D to ensure that the general population was likely to consume sufficient vitamin D. The fortification of milk with vitamin D was also adopted in Europe; however, the process was not closely monitored, and in Great Britain it caused an outbreak of vitamin D intoxication, or hypercalcemia, the clinical manifestations of which are loss of appetite, lethargy, excessive thirst and polyuria, nausea and vomiting, constipation, and muscle weakness, and renal failure if the hypercalcemic state is unrecognized and prolonged. This outbreak led to the banning of the vitamin D fortification of milk in most of Europe.

In most of present-day Europe, margarine and some cereals are the commonly available vitamin D–enriched foods. Recognizing the excessive prevalence of wintertime vitamin D deficiency, the Finnish government reinstituted the vitamin $D_3$ fortification of milk in 2002. In the United States, vitamin D fortification of milk was carefully monitored for its vitamin D content through the WARF anti-rachitic line-test assay, which prevented the occurrence of hyper-calcemia as a consequence of vitamin D fortification. The promotion and consumption of vitamin D–fortified milk, vitamin D supplementation, and sensible sun exposure were the factors responsible for the near eradication of the epidemic rickets of the early 20th century.

The current reemergence of nutritional rickets among vulnerable groups of infants warrants public health initiatives and strategies. Campaigns need to highlight the relevance of vitamin D nutrition for the skeletal and general health of all age groups. Screening strategies for rickets and vitamin D deficiency—such as assessment of vitamin D status by measuring the concentration of serum 25(OH)D—among at-risk infants need to be developed and evaluated for feasibility and cost-effectiveness. From the perspective of prevention of nutritional rickets, the focus has to rely on maintaining adequate vitamin D status for both mother and infant. Sensible sun exposure, adequate vitamin D supplementation, and the availability and consumption of vitamin D–fortified foods during pregnancy and lactation are relevant for ensuring an adequate vitamin D concentration in breast-milk. A targeted public health campaign to guarantee that all breastfed infants are receiving adequate vitamin D supplementation and are screened and monitored for rickets during infancy will ensure the eradication of reemerging rickets.

## References

1. Severe malnutrition among young children—Georgia, January 1997–June 1999.MMWR Morb Mortal Wkly Rep. 2001;50:224–227.

2. Tomashek KM, Nesby S, Scanlon KS, et al. Nutritional rickets in Georgia. Pediatrics. 2001;107:E45. Available at: http://www.pediatrics.org/cgi/content/full/107/4/e45. Accessed July 15, 2007.

3. Kreiter SR, Schwartz RP, Kirkman HN Jr, Charlton PA, Calikoglu AS, Davenport ML. Nutritional rickets in African-American breast-fed infants. J Pediatr. 2000;137:153–157.

4. Biser-Rohrbaugh A, Hadley-Miller N. Vitamin D deficiency in breast-fed toddlers. J Pediatr Orthop. 2001;21: 508–511.

5. Weisberg P, Scanlon KS, Li R, Cogswell ME. Nutritional rickets among children in the United States: review of cases reported between 1986 and 2003. Am J Clin Nutr. 2004;80:1697S–1705S.

6. Ladhani S, Srinivasan L, Buchanan C, Allgrove J. Presentation of vitamin D deficiency. Arch Dis Child. 2004;89: 781–784.

7. Eugster EA, Sane KS, Brown DM. Minnesota rickets: need for policy changes to support vitamin D supplementation. Minn Med. 1996;79:29–32.

8. Binet A, Kooh SW. Persistence of vitamin D deficiency rickets in Toronto in the 1990s. Can J Public Health. 1996; 87:227–230.

9. Holick MF. Resurrection of vitamin D deficiency and rickets. J Clin Invest. 2006;116:2062–2072.

10. Institute of Medicine. *Dietary Reference Intakes for Calcium, Phosphorus, Magnesium, Vitamin D, and Fluoride.* Washington, DC: National Academy Press; 1997;251–287.

11. Vitamins: vitamin D. In: Kleinman RE, ed. *Pediatric Nutrition Handbook.* 4th ed. Elk Grove Village, Ill: American Academy of Pediatrics; 1998:275–277.

12. Hollis BW, Wagner CL. Vitamin D requirements during lactation: high-dose maternal supplementation as therapy to prevent hypovitaminosis D for both the mother and nursing infant. Am J Clin Nutr. 2004;80:1752S–1758S.

13. Rajakumar K, Thomas SB. Reemerging nutritional rickets: a historical perspective.Arch Pediatr Adolesc Med. 2005;159:335–341.

14. Holick MF. Vitamin D: the under-appreciated D-lightful hormone that is important for skeletal and cellular health. Curr Opin Endocrinol Diabetes. 2002;9: 87–98.

15. Holick MF. McCollum Award Lecture, 1994: vitamin D—new horizons for the 21st century. Am J Clin Nutr. 1994; 60:619–630.

16. Stamp TCB, Round JM. Seasonal changes in human plasma levels of 25 (OH) vitamin D. Nature. 1974;247: 563–565.

17. McLauglin M, Fairney A, Lester E, et al. Seasonal variations in serum 25-hydroxycholecalciferol in healthy people. Lancet. 1974;i:536–537.

18. Webb AR, Kline L, Holick MF. Influence of season and latitude on the cutaneous synthesis of vitamin $D_3$: exposure to winter sunlight in Boston and Edmonton will not promote vitamin $D_3$ synthesis in human skin. J Clin Endocrinol Metab. 1988;67:1108–1110.

19. Holick MF, MacLaughlin JA, Clark MB, et al. Photosynthesis of previtamin D3 in human skin and the physiologic consequences. Science. 1980;210: 203–205.

20. Norman AW. Sunlight, season, skin pigmentation, vitamin D, and 25-hydroxy vitamin D: integral component of vitamin D endocrine system. Am J Clin Nutr. 1998;67:1108–1110.

21. Harris SS, Dawson-Hughes B. Seasonal changes in plasma 25-hydroxyvitamin D concentrations in young American black and white women. Am J Clin Nutr. 1998;67:1232–1236.

22. Clemens TL, Henderson SL, Adams JS, et al. Increased skin pigment reduces the capacity of skin to synthesise vitamin $D_3$. Lancet. 1982;1:74–76.

23. Nesby-O'Dell S, Scanlon KS, Cogswell ME, et al. Hypovitaminosis D prevalence and determinants among African American and white women of reproductive age: third National Nutrition Examination Survey, 1988–1994. Am J Clin Nutr. 2002;76:187–192.

24. Moore CE, Murphy MM, Holick MF. Vitamin D intakes by children and adults in the United States differ among ethnic groups. J Nutr. 2005;135: 2478–2485.

25. American Academy of Pediatrics. Prevention of rickets and vitamin D deficiency: new guidelines for vitamin D intake. Pediatrics. 2003;111:908–910.